Tainá Luana V. L. Zuchi
Luciana Corassa
Gustavo Bonetto

Ehrlichiosis, babesiosis and canine leishmaniasis

Tainá Luana V. L. Zuchi
Luciana Corassa
Gustavo Bonetto

Ehrlichiosis, babesiosis and canine leishmaniasis

Evaluation of the occurrence of Ehrlichia canis,
Babesia canis and Leishmania infantum in dogs
in the municipality of Concórdia-SC

This book is a translation from the original published under ISBN 978-613-9-77629-0.

Publisher:
Sciencia Scripts
is a trademark of
Dodo Books Indian Ocean Ltd. and OmniScriptum S.R.L publishing group

120 High Road, East Finchley, London, N2 9ED, United Kingdom
Str. Armeneasca 28/1, office 1, Chisinau MD-2012, Republic of Moldova, Europe
Printed at: see last page
ISBN: 978-620-6-58873-3

SUMMARY

SUMMARY

Canine ehrlichiosis, canine babesiosis and canine leishmaniasis are vector-borne diseases with a high incidence in many countries around the world. The causative agent of canine *ehrlichiosis* is *Ehrlichia canis,* while *Leishmania infantum* causes canine visceral leishmaniasis. Both are intracellular parasites, with *E. canis* being transmitted by the tick *Rhiphicephalus sanguineus* and *L. infantum* by the phlebotomine *Lutzomyia longipalpis.* Babesiosis is another disease caused by haemoparasites, the protozoa of the large *Babesia* spp family, which can also be transmitted by the *R. sanguineus* tick. Diseases caused by haemoparasites can trigger similar clinical and laboratory changes in the host, which can lead to conflicts when it comes to diagnosis. And often, because they share vectors, the animals could be co-infected. In addition, leishmaniasis is a zoonosis that is very harmful to human health. The aim of this study was to assess the occurrence of these diseases in the municipality of Concórdia, in the west of Santa Catarina. To this end, blood was collected from 370 animals treated at the Clinical Practice Centre of the Instituto Federal Catarinense (IFC) - Concórdia, as well as at clinics in the city. Antibodies were tested using the Indirect Immunofluorescence Reaction (IIFR) for *L. infantum,* ELISA for *B. canis* and for *E. canis.* The Chi-square test at a significance level of 5% was used to compare positive and negative animals within the sample population. Of the 370 samples evaluated, 55 (14.86%) were positive for leishmaniasis, 159 (42.97%) for ehrlichiosis and 158 (42.70%) for babesiosis. Of the 55 samples positive for leishmaniasis, 9 (16.36%) had co-infection with ehrlichiosis, 17 (30.90%) with babesiosis and 10 (18.18%) for both diseases. Among the variables analysed, only for ehrlichiosis was there a statistically significant difference in location, access to the street and race (p= 0.00001; p= 0.0005 and p= 0.0205 respectively). The other diseases showed no statistically significant difference. Of the 370 samples, 191 were randomly selected and submitted to the Polymerase Chain Reaction (PCR) test for the three agents. Of these, only 4.19 per cent were positive for babesiosis. These results suggest that all three diseases are present in the municipality of Concórdia, although leishmaniasis requires studying the presence of the vector in the municipality. Furthermore, the co-infection of ehrlichiosis and babesiosis with leishmaniasis reinforces the assumption that the *R. sanguineus* tick is a possible vector for *L. infantum.*

CHAPTER 1

INTRODUCTION

Canine ehrlichiosis

Ehrlichiosis is caused by *E. canis*, an obligate intracellular gram-negative bacterium (DUMLER et al., 2001), transmitted mainly by the tick *Rhiphicephalus sanguineus* (LEWIS et al., 1977). The disease has an incubation period of eight to 20 days (NEER and HARRUS, 2006) and after this period, the acute, subclinical and chronic phases of the disease follow (HARRUS et al., 1999; WANER et al., 1999). The acute phase lasts for two to four weeks (NEER and HARRUS, 2006) and is characterised by hyperthermia, weight loss, anorexia, pale mucous membranes, depression, lymphadenomegaly, splenomegaly, hepatomegaly, cardiorespiratory disorders, haemorrhagic diathesis, vasculitis, ocular and muscular signs and polyarthritis (NEER and HARRUS 2006; WANER et al., 1999). Other authors have also observed melena, epistaxis, oedema, renal sensitivity, vomiting and diarrhoea (FARIA, RIBEIRO and TINUCCI-COSTA, 2003).

The subclinical phase lasts from months to years (NEER & HARRUS, 2006). The animal may have persistent thrombocytopenia and leucopenia, but with no clinical signs (WANER et al., 1997; HARRUS et al., 1998). In this phase, antibody titres persist in the serum for more than six months, indicating a prolonged duration of infection and antigenic stimulation (WANER et al., 1997; HARRUS et al., 1998).

Dogs, unable to mount an effective immune response against the bacteria, become chronically infected (HARRUS et al., 1998). At this stage, dogs may show generalised organ damage (HARRUS et al., 1999).

ELISA is a simple test for detecting antibodies against *E. canis* and is useful for monitoring antibody levels, especially in the sub-clinical and chronic phases of the disease (BABO-TERRA, 2004 apud SILVA, 2015).

Canine Babesiosis

Canine babesiosis is caused by the protozoa *Babesia canis* and *Babesia gibsoni*, which parasitise the host's erythrocytes, causing haemolytic anaemia and significant systemic involvement in the animal (AYOOB et al., 2010). Babesia are transmitted by ticks, with *B. canis vogeli* and *B. gibsoni* being transmitted by the *R. sanguineus* tick (AYOOB et al., 2010), which is commonly found in Brazil (LABRUNA and PEREIRA, 2001). There is also vertical and horizontal transmission and transmission through blood transfusions (AYOOB et al., 2010).

The clinical presentation of babesiosis can vary from hyperacute to subclinical (TABOADA and LOBETTI, 2006; AYOOB et al., 2010). Hyperacute infection is rare and is characterised by a high mortality rate due to extensive tissue damage (FREEMAN et al., 1994). However, the acute phase is the most common clinical presentation, characterised by haemolytic anaemia, fever, lethargy, splenomegaly, lymphadenomegaly and thrombocytopenia (JACOBSON et al., 1994; TABOADA and LOBETTI, 2006). According to Jacobson et al. (1994) chronic infection can occur, although it is not well characterised. Some animals can remain in the subclinical phase, especially when infected with *B. canis vogeli* and *B. gibsoni* (MACINTIRE et al., 2002).

Babesiosis can be diagnosed in situations of low parasitaemia using the ELISA test (OLICHESKI, 2003, apud PINTO, R. L., 2009). However, differentiating between cases of previous exposure and active infection may not be possible by assessing serological titres (TRAPP et al., 2006).

Canine visceral leishmaniasis

Leishmaniasis is an infectious disease that affects humans, domestic and wild animals and is caused by obligate intracellular protozoa belonging to the genus *Leishmania* (BANETH and GALLEGO, 2012). The vectors involved in the transmission of leishmaniasis are insects called phlebotomines, among which *Lutzomyia longipalpis* and *Lutzomyia cruzi* are found in Brazil (FEITOSA, 2006).

Three forms of presentation are recognised: visceral, cutaneous and mucocutaneous. Among these forms of presentation, the most important in the canine species is visceral leishmaniasis, caused by *Leishmania infantum* (BANETH and GALLEGO, 2012). Domestic dogs are the main reservoir of the parasite and play an important role in the transmission of the disease (CASTRO-JUNIOR et al., 2014), both because of their proximity to humans and because many dogs are positive and asymptomatic, and act as carriers of the parasite, being a source of contamination for the vectors that transmit the disease (MARZOCHI et al., 2009).

According to Perego et al. (2014), the main alterations on clinical examination are crusted lesions on the skin, especially in the ear, muzzle and periorbital regions, as well as furfuraceous scaling and multifocal alopecia. What can be observed is that animals with dermatological alterations usually also have systemic involvement, as the parasites need to be disseminated throughout the body to cause skin lesions (SILVA, 2007). Weight loss with normal or increased appetite, polyuria, polydipsia, muscle wasting, depression, vomiting, diarrhoea, coughing, epistaxis, sneezing and melena can also be observed (NELSON and COUTO, 2006). Splenomegaly, generalised lymphadenopathy, fever, rhinitis, increased lung noise, jaundice, tender and swollen joints are also common on clinical examination (LAPPIN, 2004).

Serological tests such as the indirect immunofluorescence reaction (RIFI) are widely used to detect the disease in epidemiological surveys (ALVES; BEVILACQUA, 2004 *apud* MORAIS, 2013*)*. Polymerase chain reaction (PCR) assays are also used to diagnose the disease and have high sensitivity and specificity, as they detect the presence of the parasite's DNA in blood and tissues (GALLEGO et al., 2009).

Santa Catarina was considered a disease-free state until the first half of 2010, when the first five cases were reported and confirmed in the municipality of Florianópolis (FIGUEIREDO et al., 2012). In the western region of the state, the first confirmed case was in the municipality of Chapecó, in August this year (DIRETORIA DE VIGILÂNCIA EPIDEMIOLÓGICA, 2017). In the same month, the first human case was also confirmed in the municipality of Florianópolis (PREFEITURA MUNICIPAL DE FLORIANÓPOLIS, 2017).

Given the importance of these diseases, this study assessed their occurrence in animals treated at the Clinical Practice Centre of the IFC - Concórdia - SC, as well as in veterinary clinics and rural areas of the city.

CHAPTER 2

MATERIAL AND METHODS

Experimental Animals

A total of 370 dogs were used in this study. Of these samples, all were used in the evaluation for canine ehrlichiosis, canine leishmaniasis and canine babesiosis. Of the 370 samples, 191 were chosen at random and submitted to the Polymerase Chain Reaction (PCR) assay for the three agents. The dogs used in the study were those showing clinical alterations compatible with haemoparasites, or asymptomatic, treated at the Clinical Practices Centre of the IFC-Concórdia-SC, private clinics and in rural areas of the city. From each dog, 5 mL of whole blood was collected and desorbed, and the serum used to detect *anti-E. canis, anti-B. canis* and *anti-L. infantum* antibodies. Among the animals collected, information was collected on their sex, access to the street, place of residence, age and breed. All this information was then correlated with the serological results (SILVA et al., 2013). The samples collected were stored in the Clinical Analyses Laboratory at IFC Concórdia at -20°C until they were used.

ELISA for the detection of *E. canis* antibodies

An ELISA test was used to detect *E. canis* antibodies using a kit marketed by the Imunodot laboratory (Imunotest®) for *E. canis,* and the reaction was carried out according to the manufacturer's instructions. The reactions took place in the Clinical Analyses Laboratory at IFC-Concórdia. To carry out the test, the plates sensitised with total *E. canis* antigen were previously removed from the refrigerator and left at room temperature for 10 minutes. Next, 100 µl of the negative and positive control sera were added to the corresponding wells and 100 µl of the test samples diluted (5:1000), recording the position of each one as marked on the microplates, except in holes H2, H4, H6, H8, H10 and H12. The plates were incubated for 1 hour in a humid chamber at 37°C. At the end of incubation, the plates were washed three times with PBS-Tween 20 and dried on a flat surface padded with layers of paper towels. Then 100 µl/well of the diluted conjugate was added and incubated again for 1 hour at 37 °C in a humid chamber. At the end, the washing and drying procedure was repeated, 100 µl of the substrate solution was added and then the plate was wrapped in aluminium foil and incubated at room temperature for 45 minutes. Then 50 pl/well of the reaction stop solution was added. Finally, the plates were read on an ELISA reader with a 405nm filter. To interpret the results, the cut-off index was calculated (average optical density of the negative control serum multiplied by 2.5). Samples that showed an intense yellow colour and an optical density greater than or equal to the cut-off index were considered positive for *E. canis, while* samples that did not show a yellow colour and an optical density greater than or equal to the cut-off index were considered positive for *E. canis.*

had an intense yellow colour and an optical density lower than the cut-off index were considered negative for the agent in question.

ELISA for the detection of antibodies to *Babesia canis vogeli*

The ELISA test *was used* to detect anti-B. *canis* antibodies using kits marketed by the Imunodot laboratory (Imunotest®) for *B. canis,* and the reaction was carried out according to the manufacturer's instructions. The reactions took place in the Clinical Analyses Laboratory at IFC-Concórdia. To carry out the test, the plates sensitised with total *B. canis* antigen were previously removed from the refrigerator and left at room temperature for 10 minutes. Then 100 µl of the negative and positive control sera were added to the corresponding wells and 100 pl of the test samples diluted (5:1000), recording the position of each one as marked on the microplates, except in holes H2, H4, H6, H8, H10 and H12. The plates were incubated for 1 hour in a humid chamber at 37°C. At the end of incubation, the plates were washed three times with PBS-Tween 20 and dried on a flat surface padded with layers of paper towels. Then 100 µl/well of the diluted conjugate was added and incubated again for 1 hour at 37 °C in a humid chamber. At the end, the washing and drying procedure was repeated and 100 pl of the substrate solution was added, after which the plate was wrapped in aluminium foil and incubated at room temperature for 45 minutes. Then 50 pl/well of the reaction stop solution was added. Finally, the plates were read on an ELISA reader with a 405nm filter. To interpret the results, the cut-off index was calculated (average optical density of the negative control serum multiplied by 2.5). Samples that showed an intense yellow colour and an optical density greater than or equal to the cut-off index were considered positive for *B. canis, while* samples that did not show an intense yellow colour and an optical density lower than the cut-off index were considered negative for the agent in question.

Indirect Immunofluorescence Reaction (IIFR) to detect *anti-Leishmania infantum* antibodies

The Indirect Immunofluorescence Reaction (IIFR) was carried out at the Clinical Analyses Laboratory of the Federal Institute of Santa Catarina. To carry out the RIFI, kits marketed by the company Imunodot (Imunotest®) for *L. infantum were* purchased. The sera, individually diluted 1:40 in sterile saline solution, were added briefly to the slides containing the antigen. The slides were then incubated for 30 minutes at 37 °C in a humid chamber. The slides were then washed in PBS and after drying, the conjugate (dog anti-IgG, labelled with fluorescein isothiocyanate) was added, diluted 1:30 in PBS containing 1mg of Evans blue. The slides were incubated in a humid chamber, washed, dried and mounted in buffered glycerine. Reading was carried out under an inverted light/fluorescence microscope and the greenish fluorescence of the parasites on the entire surface was considered positive and the reaction negative when there was no fluorescence. A positive and a negative control serum were used on each slide with 10 tests.

DNA Extraction and Polymerase Chain Reaction (PCR)

For DNA extraction, the *PureLink® Genomic DNA Mini Kit,* marketed by Invitrogen™, was purchased, using 200 µL of whole blood to carry out the extraction. The material resulting from the extraction was eluted in 50 µl of ultrapure water free of DNAse and RNAse and stored at - 20°C until use. The positive and negative controls of the reactions were subjected to the same extraction protocol as the samples tested. The PCR for ehrlichiosis used the primers EHR 16SD with the sequence 5'-GGTACCYACAGAAGAAGTCC-3' and EHR 16SR with the sequence 5'-TAGCACTCATCGTTTACAGC-3', this sequencing being recommended by Harrus et al. (2011). For babesiosis, primers BAB143-167 with the sequence 5'-CCGTGCTAATTGTAGGCTAATACA-3' and BAB694-667 with the sequence 5'- GCTTGAAACACTCTARTTTCTCAAAG- 3' were used. This sequencing was used by Almeida (2011). For leishmaniasis, we used the primers LEISH1 with the sequence 5'- GGCCCACTATATTACACCAACCCC-3' and LEISH2 with the sequence 5'- GGGGTAGGGGCGTTCTGCGAA- 3'. This sequencing was used by Passos et al. (1996). These oligonucleotides are shown in Table 1 below.

Table 1- Oligonucleotides used for the *E. canis* amplification reactions, *B. canis* and *L. infantum.*

Oligonucleotide Sequence 5' - 3'		*Amplicon* (bp)	Reference
EHR 16SD	GGTACCYACAGAAGTCC	345	Harrus et al.
EHR 16SR	TAGCACTCATCGTTTACAGC		(2011)
BAB143-167	CCGTGCTAATTGTAGGGCTAATACA	551	Almeida
BAB694-667	GCTTGAAACACTCTARTTTTCTCAA AG		(2011)
LEISH1	GGCCCACTATATTACACCAACCCC	120	Passos et al.
LEISH2	GGGGTAGGGGCGTTCTGCGAA		(1996)

To carry out the reaction, a total of 1 µl of the extracted DNA sample was amplified in a final volume of 25 µl, containing a buffer solution (20 mM Tris - HCl pH 8.4 and 50 mM KCl), 200 µM of dNTP, 20 pmol of each oligonucleotide and 1U of Taq polymerase. MgCl2 was also added at a final concentration of 1.0, 1.5 or 2.0 mM for the amplification reactions of Ehrlichia canis, Babesia canis or Leishmania infantum, respectively.

The PCR amplification cycles were carried out on the T100TM Thermal Cycler (BIORAD) and are described below: for *Ehrlichia* they were 95°C/3 min followed by 33 cycles of 95°C/30 sec, 53°C/30 sec and 72°C/45 sec and a final extension step 72°C/5 min; for *Babesia canis* they were 95°C/5 min followed by 35 cycles of 95°C/30 sec, 58°C/30 sec and 72°C/30 sec and a final extension step 72°C/7 min and for *Leishmania infantum* they were 94°C/3 min followed by 34 cycles of 94°C/30 sec, 55°C/30 sec and 72°C/30 sec and a final extension step 72°C/10 min. The PCR products were subjected to electrophoresis on a 1% agarose gel, stained with ethidium bromide and visualised using a transluminator (LTB-STi UV Transilluminator/ L-PIX STi-Loccus Photodocumenter).

Statistical analysis

The Chi-square test at a significance level of 5 per cent was used to compare the variables (sex, access to the street, place of residence, age and race) of the positive animals with the negative ones within the sample population, using

Minitab statistical software® 18.

CHAPTER 3

RESULTS

Of the 370 samples evaluated, 55 (14.86%) were positive for leishmaniasis, 159 (42.97%) for ehrlichiosis and 158 (42.70%) for babesiosis. Of the 55 samples positive for leishmaniasis, 9 (16.36%) had co-infection with ehrlichiosis, 17 (30.90%) with babesiosis and 10 (18.18%) for both diseases. Of the 159 samples positive for ehrlichiosis, 62 (38.75%) had co-infection with babesiosis. Among the 370 animals, 228 (61.62%) were female and 142 (38.37%) were male. Among the breeds, there were 204 (55.13%) SRDs, 40 (10.81%) poodles, 19 (5.13%) pinschers and 107 (28.93%) other breeds, such as shih tzu, German shepherd, boxer and lhasa apso. In terms of age, 21 (5.67%) animals were less than 1 year old, 136 (36.75%) were between 1 and 5 years old, 105 (28.37%) were between 5 and 10 years old, 85 (22.97%) were over 10 years old and 23 (6.21%) had no age information. As for location, 297 (80.27%) came from urban areas, 73 (19.72%) from rural areas. With regard to access to the street, 225 (60.81%) had no access and 145 (39.18%) had access.

Of the 159 dogs positive for ehrlichiosis, 91 (57.5%) were females and 68 (42.5%) were males, with no statistically significant difference (p= 0.1318). As for location, 105 (66.03%) came from urban areas and 54 (33.96%) from rural areas. In this respect, there was a statistically significant difference (p=0.00001), so there is a positive correlation between seropositivity and living in an urban area. With regard to access to the street, 81 (50.94%) had no access and 78 (49.05%) had access, and there was also a statistically significant difference (p= 0.0005) in this respect. With regard to breed, there were 93 (58.49%) SRDs, 9 (5.66%) poodles, 6 (3.77%) pinschers as well as 6

(3.77%) German shepherds and 45 (28.30%) other breeds. There was a statistically significant difference between the breed of animal and seropositivity (p= 0.0205). With regard to age, 8 (5.03%) dogs were less than 1 year old, 65 (40.88%) were between 1 and 5 years old, 43 (27.04%) were between 5 and 10 years old, 32 (20.12%) were over 10 years old and 11 (6.91%) had no age information. There was no statistically significant difference between age and seropositivity (p= 0.3913). The data is shown in Table 2 below.

Table 2. Seropositivity of dogs to ELISA for *anti-E. canis* antibodies in the municipality of Concórdia, Santa Catarina.

Variables	Dogs		p-value[a]
	Positive (n°/%)	Negative (n°/%)	
Females	91/159 (57,5%)	137/211 (64,93%)	0,1318
Males	68/159 (42,5%)	74/211 (35,07%)	
Urban area	105/159 (66,03%)	192/211 (90,99%)	0,00001
Rural areas	54/159 (33,96%)	19/211 (9,01%)	
With street access	78/159 (49,05%)	66/211 (31,28%)	0,0005
No access to the street	81/159 (50,94%)	145/211 (68,72%)	
SRD	93/159 (58,49%)	111/211 (52,61%)	
Poodle	9/159 (5,66%)	31/211 (14,70%)	
Pinscher	6/159 (3,77%)	12/211 (5,69%)	0,0205
German Shepherd	6/159 (3,77%)	2/211 (0,94%)	
Other breeds	45/159 (28,30%)	55/211 (26,06%)	
Less than 1 year	8/159 (5,03%)	12/211 (5,69%)	
Between 1 and 5 years	65/159 (40,88%)	71/211 (33,65%)	
Between 5 and 10 years	43/159 (27,04%)	56/211 (26,54)	0,3913
Over 10 years old	32/159 (20,12%)	60/211 (28,44%)	
Age not stated	11/159 (6.91%)	12/211 (5,69%)	

[a] 5% significance level.

For babesiosis, among the 158 seropositive animals, 57 (35.84%) were males and 101 (64.15%) were females, with no statistically significant difference (p= 0.3802). As for location, 136 (83.54%) came from urban areas and 26 (16.45%) from rural areas and there was no statistically significant difference (p= 0.1389). With regard to access to the street, 98 (62.02%) had no access and 60 (37.97%) had access, and there was no statistically significant difference (p= 0.6795). With regard to breed, 83 (52.53%) were SRDs, 17 (10.75%) were poodles, 7 (4.43%) were pinschers and 51 (32.27%) were mixed breeds. There was no statistically significant difference between breed and seropositivity (p= 0.6408). With regard to age, 5 (3.16%) were less than a year old, 60 (37.97%) were between 1 and 5 years old, 44 (27.84%) were between 5 and 10 years old, 35 (22.15%) were over 10 years old and 14 (8.86%) had no age information. There was also no statistically significant difference between age and seropositivity (p= 0.1721). The data is shown in Table 3 below.

Table 3. Seropositivity of dogs to ELISA for *anti-B. canis* antibodies in the municipality of Concórdia, Santa Catarina.

Variables	Dogs		p-value[a]
	Positive (n/%)	**Negative (n/%)**	
Females	101/158 (64,15%)	126/213 (59,15%)	0,3802
Males	57/158 (35,84%)	87/213 (40,85%)	
Urban area	136/158 (83,54%)	165/213 (77,46%)	0,1389
Rural areas	26/158 (16,45%)	47/213 (22,54%)	
With street access	60/158 (37,97%)	85/213 (39,91%)	0,6795
No access to the street	98/158 (62,02%)	127/213 (60,09%)	
SRD	83/158 (52,53%)	121/213 (56,81%)	
Poodle	17/158 (10,75%)	23/213 (10,80%)	0,6408
Pinscher	7/158 (4,43%)	12/213 (5,63%)	
Other breeds	51/158 (32,27%)	56/213 (26,29%)	
Less than 1 year	5/158 (3,16%)	16/213 (7,51%)	
Between 1 and 5 years	60/158 (37,97)	76/213 (35,68%)	
Between 5 and 10 years	44/158 (27,84%)	61/213 (28,64%)	0,1721
Over 10 years old	35/158 (22,15%)	50/213 (23,47%)	
Age not stated	14/158 (8,86%)	9/213 (4,22%)	

[a] 5% significance level.

Of the 55 animals positive for leishmaniasis, 21 (38.18%) were males and 34 (61.81%) were females, with no statistically significant difference (p= 0.9740). As for location, 45 (81.81%) came from urban areas and 10 (18.18%) from rural areas, with no statistically significant difference between location and seropositivity (0.7545). With regard to access to the street, 39 (70.90%) had no access and 16 (29.9%) had access. There was no statistically significant difference between access to the street and seropositive animals (p= 0.096). In terms of breed, 34 (61.81%) were SRDs, 5 (9.05%) were poodles, 3 (5.45%) were pinschers and 13 (23.69%) were other breeds such as Yorkshire and German Shepherd, with no statistically significant difference (p= 0.7372). As for age, no animal was less than a year old, 23 (41.81%) were between 1 and 5 years old, 15 (27.27%) were between 5 and 10 years old, 15 (27.27%) were over 10 years old and 2 (3.6%) had no reported age, with no statistically significant difference (p= 0.5242). The data is shown in Table 4 below and Figure 1 shows one of the seroreactive samples for leishmaniasis.

Table 4 - Seropositivity of dogs to the Indirect Immunofluorescence Reaction (IIFR) for *anti-L. infantum* antibodies in the municipality of Concórdia, Santa Catarina, Brazil

Variables	Dogs		*p-value* a
	Positive (n/%)	Negative (n/%)	
Females	34/55 (61,81%)	194/315 (61,59%)	0,9740
Males	21/55 (38,18%)	121/315 (38,41%)	
Urban area	45/55 (81,81%)	252/315 (80%)	0,7545
Rural areas	10/55 (18,18%)	63/315 (20%)	
With street access	16/55 (29,9%)	129/315 (40,95%)	0,096
No access to the street	39/55 (70,90%)	186/315 (59,05%)	
SRD	34/55 (61,81%)	170/315 (53,97%)	
Poodle	5/55 (9,05%)	35/315 (11,11%)	0,7370
Pinscher	3/55 (5,45%)	17/315 (5,40%)	
Other breeds	13/55 (23,69%)	93/315 (29,52%)	
Less than 1 year	0	19/315 (6,03%)	
Between 1 and 5 years	23/55 (41,81%)	113/315 (35,87%)	
Between 5 and 10 years	15/55 (27,27%)	92/315 (29,21%)	0,5242
Over 10 years old	15/55 (27,27%)	70/315 (22,22%)	
Age not stated	2/55 (3,6%)	21/315 (6,66%)	

a 5% significance level.

Figure 1- Indirect immunofluorescence reaction using antigen from promastigote forms of *Leishmania infantum.*
A: Positive control. B: Negative control. C: Reagent sample.

Of the 191 samples used for PCR analysis, 43.45% (83/191) were considered positive for ehrlichiosis, 43.98% (84/191) positive for babesiosis and 14.66% (28/191) for leishmaniasis. In addition, 4.19% (8/191) were seropositive for all three diseases. However, only 4.19% (8/191) of the samples were positive for babesiosis by PCR (figure 2). All the samples were negative for ehrlichiosis and leishmaniasis. Of the 8 babesiosis PCR-positive animals, 2 (25%) were males and 6 females (75%), 3 (37.5%) from rural areas and 5 (62.50%) from urban areas, 4 (50%) with access to the street and 4 (50%) without access, 1 (12.50%) pinscher and 7 (87.50%) SRD and finally, in terms of age, no animal was less than 1 year old, 5 (62.50%) were between 1 and 5 years old, 1 (12.50%) were between 5 and 10 years old and 2 (25%) were over 10 years old. These data were not statistically analysed due to the low number of positive samples. Figure 2 shows the test-positive samples.

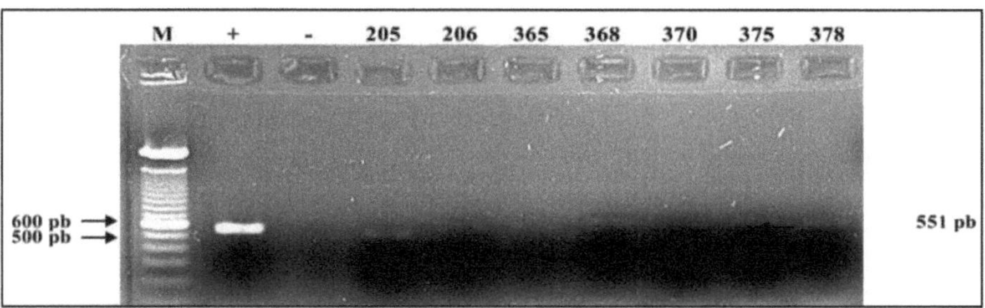

Figure 2- Polymerase Chain Reaction with DNA samples tested for *Babesia canis* visualised on a 1.0% agarose gel.
"M": 100 bp molecular marker; "+": Positive Control, "-": Negative Control, in the sequence the numbering identifies the sample tested. The arrow labelled "551 bp" indicates the

presence of amplification of a specific product.

CHAPTER 4

DISCUSSION

This study found that 14.86% (55/370) of the animals tested showed antibodies to *L. infantum*. This result suggests that the disease occurs in Concórdia and serves as a warning, because if there is an outbreak of the transmitting agent, the municipality will be at risk of transmitting the disease between dogs and humans. In addition, seropositivity for ehrlichiosis was 43.24 per cent (160/370) and for babesiosis 42.97 per cent (159/370). This suggests that both diseases are endemic in the municipality.

According to Boraschi and Nunes (2007), most Brazilian states have had cases of visceral leishmaniasis. Complementing this information, an epidemiological study carried out in the city of Jaciara-MT detected a prevalence of 35.6% among 7,545 dogs tested (BRITO et al., 2014). In Minas Gerais, 30.2% of the 16,529 dogs analysed were positive (BARATA et al., 2013). In the state of Tocantins, Morais et al. (2013) showed that of 111 dogs tested, 51.35% were infected. In the state of Rio de Janeiro, Silva et al. (2013) analysed 524 dogs suspected of having leishmaniasis and found that 28.24% were positive. In the same study, the authors showed a prevalence of approximately 60% in the city of Seropédica. Maziero et al. (2014) carried out a study of 252 animals in the west of the state of Santa Catarina and 43 of them were seropositive for *L. infantum* using the Indirect Immunofluorescence Reaction (IIFR) test. The author also suggested that the region is exposed to the agent in question, which is in line with this survey. Another piece of data that reinforces the suggestion that the western region is exposed to the agent is the case of canine leishmaniasis confirmed in the city of Chapecó (DIRETORIA DE VIGILÂNCIA EPIDEMIOLÓGICA, 2017).

In the southern region, the first cases of leishmaniasis were recorded in

2008, in São Borja - RS, where the first human case also occurred (FIGUEIREDO et al., 2012). In Paraná, Tomaz-Soccol et al. (2009) analysed 24 animals and isolated the parasite in 19 of them. In Santa Catarina, the first cases were notified and confirmed in 2010, in the municipality of Florianópolis (FIGUEIREDO et. al., 2012).

Most animals seropositive for leishmaniasis are asymptomatic (BARATA et al., 2013; PENAFORTE et al., 2013). Castro Junior et al. (2014) showed that of 400 positive dogs, 65.6% were asymptomatic. These results reinforce the importance of the dog as a domestic reservoir of *Leishmania infantum* (SILVA, 2007), which can live with the parasite for long periods without developing the clinical disease, contributing to the maintenance of the disease (BARATA et al., 2013). The study reported here reinforces this information, since 100% of the seropositive animals had no clinical signs consistent with the disease.

As for location, 10 (18.18%) of the animals came from rural areas and 45 (81.81%) from urban areas, with no statistical difference (p= 0.7545). The prevalence of seropositive animals in urban areas is possibly due to the process of urbanisation of the disease (TOMAZ-SOCCOL, et al. 2009).

With regard to gender, 21 (38.18%) of the animals were male and 34 (61.81%) were female, with no statistically significant difference (p= 0.9740). This is in line with the results of studies carried out in Paraná by Constantino et al. (2014), who also found no statistically significant difference between seropositivity and gender.

A study carried out in Bahia using the ELISA test identified 72 out of 200 dogs seropositive for ehrlichiosis, which represented 36% of the animals (CARLOS, et al., 2007). Using the same serological test, another study obtained similar results, with 46.67% seropositivity in Pernambuco (BORBA et al., 2002, apud CARLOS, et al., 2007). Likewise, Vieira et al. (2013) found that 62 of the 138 dogs sampled in their study were positive for ehrlichiosis using the same test. In the present survey, using ELISA, 159 of the 370 (42.97%) animals were positive for ehrlichiosis, which is in line with the other studies cited.

Labarthe et al. (2003) analysed 2553 dogs using ELISA and found that 505 animals were serologically positive for *E. canis, of* which 274 were males and 226 were females. In the present study, of the 160 seropositive animals, 68 were males and 92 were females, which is in line with Labarthe et al. (2003), since females were more seropositive in both. Also, in a study carried out by Carvalho et al. (2008), they reported that when assessing the gender variable there was no statistically significant difference (p> 0.26), as in the present study.

Studies carried out in Brazil have shown that the seroprevalence of ehrlichiosis in dogs varied according to region; for example, 31.2 per cent in northern Brazil, 42.5 per cent in central Brazil, 35.6 per cent in the northeast, 44.7 per cent in the southeast and 4.8 per cent in the south (Aguiar et al., 2007; Souza et al., 2010; Silva et al., 2010; Saito et al., 2008, apud Melo et al., 2011), 2007; Souza et al., 2010; Silva et al., 2010; Costa et al., 2007; Saito et al., 2008, apud Melo et al., 2011).In the aforementioned study, carried out in the southern region by Saito et al. (2008), out of 389 dogs, only 19 (4.8%) were positive for *E. canis*. Another study by Labarthe et al. (2003) also showed a low prevalence of *E. canis* in the southern region, with 4.7 % in Paraná, 1.7 % in Rio Grande do Sul and 0.7 % in Santa Catarina, a disparity with the present study, which found a seroprevalence of 42.97 % of animals.

Studies have reported the cross-reactivity of *E. canis* with other haemoparasites, leading to false positive or false negative results, and further studies are needed to evaluate these results. Bélanger et al. (2002) showed that rapid serodiagnostic tests do not differentiate between infections by *E. canis, Ehrlichia ewingii* and *Ehrlichia chaffeensis* because these species have certain cross-reactive antigens. Cross-reaction with *Ehrlichia risticcii* (*Neoricketsia risticii*) and *Anaplasma platys has also* been demonstrated (NEER et al., 2002 apud SOUSA, 2012).

In tropical and subtropical areas, *R. sanguineus* is prevalent throughout the year (LOULY 2006, apud DANTAS-TORRES 2010). The southern region of Brazil has a subtropical climate and the four seasons are well defined (SANTA CATARINA, 1986 apud CERON 2014), thus representing an ideal climate for tick prevalence. Therefore, the tick is considered to be well adapted to the region's environment, based on the relatively high rate of seropositive animals for ehrlichiosis and babesiosis in this study.

In this survey, there was a prevalence of seropositive animals from urban areas, corroborating Vieira et al. (2013), who found 44 animals from urban areas and 18 from rural areas, out of a total of 138 dogs serologically tested by ELISA. Furthermore, this may be due to the higher prevalence of the tick in urban areas, as mentioned by Labruna (2001), who states that the *R. sanguineus* tick is found preferentially in urban areas of the country, but in lower densities in rural areas.

The seropositivity found for babesiosis in this survey corroborates studies carried out in other regions. In the state of São Paulo Dell' Porto et al. (1993) found a prevalence of 42.4% using the Indirect Immunofluorescence (RIFI) technique. In the state of Minas Gerais Bastos et al. (2004) identified a seroprevalence of 42% among animals with suspected haemoparasitosis, and in the same state Milken et al. (2004) reported a prevalence of 51.4% using the RIFI technique. In the state of Rio de Janeiro, Vilela et al. (2013) reported a prevalence of 11.9% using the PCR technique. Trapp et al. (2006) reported seropositivity of 35.7% using the RIFI test in the state of Paraná. Based on these results, it can be suggested that the disease is endemic in the municipality of Concórdia - SC.

Of the animals seropositive for babesiosis, 85.54 per cent (136/158) came from urban areas. This result suggests that the disease is more widespread in urban areas than in rural areas, and similarly other studies have also detected this information. Krawczak et al. (2015) only analysed samples from urban animals in the state of Minas Gerais and reported a prevalence of 31.2% (30/96). In relation to animals living in rural areas, 14.46% (23/159) were positive. These results are in line with data obtained by O'Dwyer et al. (2009) who, when assessing a population of dogs from rural areas in the state of São Paulo, reported a prevalence of 8% (12/150). According to the authors, the low seropositivity of *B. canis* in rural dogs is due to the low prevalence of *R. sanguineus in* these areas*, and* the animals do not acquire immunity to the parasite.

The absence of a relationship between seropositivity and the gender variable observed in this study was also observed by Guimarães et al. (2009), since 103 of the seropositive animals were male and 114 were female, with a p-value > 0.05 in the statistical analysis. The absence of a statistically significant difference shows that males and females have the same risk of being affected by the disease.

As mentioned above, this study found co-infection between the diseases. Co-infection for babesiosis and ehrlichiosis was 16.75% of the animals (62/370), which is higher than that reported in the literature. In a study carried out by Krawczak et al. (2015), nine out of 96 animals showed co-infection using the Indirect Immunofluorescence Reaction. Fonseca et al. (2017) detected 5.6% co-infection in their study using the same serological test. Krawczak et al. (2015) also observed 4.3% (by Indirect Immunofluorescence Reaction and ELISA) of dogs positive for ehrlichiosis and leishmaniasis, and this study is in line with the aforementioned author, since co-infection between ehrlichiosis and leishmaniasis was 5.13% (19/370) of the animals.

In Campo Grande - Mato Grosso do Sul, a study by Sousa (2012) showed that some of the dogs serologically positive for leishmaniasis also had antibodies against babesiosis and ehrlichiosis. Of the 60 dogs sampled that were positive for leishmaniasis, 39 (65.0%) had co-infection with ehrlichiosis, 26 (43.33%) with babesiosis and 20 (33.33%) for both (SOUSA, 2012). In the present study, the percentage of dogs serologically positive for leishmaniasis with co-infection was lower, with 16.36% (9 dogs) co-infected with ehrlichiosis; 30.90% (17 dogs) with babesiosis and 18.18% (10 dogs) with both diseases. This is possibly due to the fact that the Campo Grande region has favourable climatic conditions for the development of vectors (SALGADO, 2006 apud SOUSA, 2012), as well as leishmaniasis having a worrying status in the state of Mato Grosso do Sul according to the State Health Department (SOUSA, 2012).

It is thought that the *R. sanguineus* tick could also be an agent that transmits leishmaniasis (COUTINHO et al., 2005). Viol et al. (2016) detected protozoan DNA in 89.4 %, 40.9 % and 33.3 % of the intestines, ovaries and salivary glands of ticks, respectively. Coutinho et al. (2005), Colombo et al. (2011), Morais et al. (2013), and Campos and Costa (2014) detected the DNA in 33 %, 50 %, 44 % and 23 % of the ticks sampled, respectively (VIOL et al. 2016). Dantas-Torres et al. (2010), when collecting 73 ticks from dogs positive for leishmaniasis in northeastern Brazil, identified nine (12.3 per cent) ticks positive for the presence of the protozoan from real-time PCR. Furthermore, this was the first study to recover *L. infantum in* the salivary glands of *R. sanguineus*. It is therefore suggested that the co-infection between the diseases obtained in this study is due to the possible role of *R. sanguineus* as a potential vector for *L. infantum*.

Antibody cross-reactions are questionable aspects when it comes to diagnosing haemoparasitoses, due to the morphological similarity between species from the same family (VARGAS HERNANDEZ, 2012). Furthermore, such reactions are not observed in molecular techniques such as nPCR (IQBAL et al., (1994), NAKAGHI et al., (2008) apud VARGAS HERNANDEZ, 2012). Serological tests such as RIFI and ELISA are not very specific, which leads to cross-reactions between haemoparasites, such as reactions between *Babesia sp.*, *Babesia gibsoni* and *Rangelia vitalli*, as well as false negative results in young animals (BOBADE et al., (1989); VARGAS HERNÁNDEZ, (2010), apud SOUSA et al., 2012). FURUTA et al. (2009) standardised and compared ELISA and RIFI tests for detecting anti-B. *canis* antibodies in naturally infected dogs in order to highlight the cross-reaction between *Babesia sp.* species. As a result, there was a higher incidence of positive dogs in the ELISA with 67% and 59% for RIFI.

For ehrlichiosis, as mentioned above, cross-reactions are also common, so species identification may not be achieved, demonstrating the importance of molecular biology techniques for this purpose (WEN et al., 1997, NEER et al., 2002, apud VARGAS HERNANDEZ (2010). As mentioned above, studies have reported the cross-reactivity of haemoparasites in serological tests.

Studies carried out in endemic areas have found through serological tests that there is no cross-reaction between ehrlichiosis, babesiosis and leishmaniasis, but rather co-infection between the diseases (OLIVEIRA, et al., 2000, KRAWCZAK, et al., 2015). This is due to the taxonomy of the pathogens, with a phylogenetic distance between them, since the genus Ehrlichia is an intracellular bacterium (DUMLER, et al., 2001, apud KRAWCZAK, et al., 2015) and Babesia and Leishmania are protozoan agents (ALMOSNY et al., 2002, apud KRAWCZAK, et al., 2015).

As for the molecular test, 4.19% (8/191) of the animals were positive for B. canis in this study, a result similar to that found by Silva et al. (2012) in Maranhão (3.33%) and by Ramos et al. (2010) in Recife (7.31%). The eight animals that tested positive had no obvious clinical signs or the presence of the vector. Five of these animals were also positive for the serological test. It is suggested that the serology-positive animals could be in the subclinical phase of the disease and the PCR-positive animals could be showing peak parasitaemia at the time of diagnosis, as concluded by Hernández et al. (2010), who found 51.6% of the animals in their study to be serology-positive and only 5.5% in the molecular test.

CHAPTER 5

CONCLUSION

This study suggests that canine visceral leishmaniasis is a disease present in the municipality of Concórdia, since dogs were found to be serologically positive for the disease. Given that canine cases precede human cases and that human infection is only possible in areas where the vector is present, there is a need to study the presence of the phlebotome in the city, as well as the possibility that the *R. sanguineus* tick is also a vector of this disease. Furthermore, due to the occurrence of serologically positive dogs, it is believed that there is a risk of new animals being infected and human cases occurring in the future, making it essential to pass on information to the population about preventing cases in dogs and humans.

As for bebesiosis and ehrlichiosis, it is suggested that both diseases occur in the municipality, as well as being more widespread in urban than rural areas, possibly due to the higher prevalence of *R. sanguineus in* these areas. In addition, those who tested positive for the molecular test could be suffering from peak parasitaemia. The co-infection of these diseases with leishmaniasis reinforces the assumption that the *R. sanguineus* tick is a possible vector for *L. infantum. In* addition, there was a prevalence of serologically positive dogs for leishmaniasis from urban areas, where the tick is better adapted.

CHAPTER 6

BIBLIOGRAPHICAL REFERENCES

ALMEIDA, A P. **Investigation of *Rickettsia, Ehrlichia, Anaplasma, Babesia, Hepatozoon* and *Leishmania* in free-living *Cerdocyonthous* dogs in the State of Espírito Santo.** 2011. 80 p. Master's thesis - University of São Paulo, São Paulo.

AYOOB, A. L. **Clinical management of canine babesiosis.** J. Vet. Emerg. Critical Care, v. 20, n. 1, p.77-89, 2010.

BANETH, G.; GALLEGO, L. Leishamaniasis. In: GREENE, C. E. **Infectious Diseases of the Dog and Cat.** In: 4th Edition. St. Louis: Saunders Elsevier, 2012, p. 734 - 746.

BARATA, R. A.; et al. **Epidemiology of Visceral Leishmaniasis in a Reemerging Focus of Intense Transmission in Minas Gerais State, Brazil.** Biomed. Res. Int., v. 2013, 6 p., 2013.

BASTOS, C.V.; Moreira S.M.; Passos L.M.F. **Retrospective Study (19982001) on Canine Babesiosis in Belo Horizonte, Minas Gerais, Brazil.** N.Y. Acad. Sci, v. 1026, p.158-160, 2004.

BÉLANGER, M., et al. **Comparison of Serological Detection Methods for Diagnosis of *Ehrlichia canis* Infections in Dogs.** Journal of Clinical Microbiology, vol. 40, n. 9, p. 3506-3508, 2002.

BORASCHI, C. S. S. & NUNES, C. M. **Epidemiological aspects of urban** visceral leishmaniasis in Brazil. Clínica Veterinária, v. 71, p. 44 - 48, 2007.

BRITO, V. N. et al. **Epidemiological aspects of visceral leishmaniasis in Jaciara, Mato Grosso, Brazil, 2003 to 2012.** Rev. Bras. Parasitol. Vet., v. 23, n. 1, p. 63-68, 2014.

CARLOS, R. S. A., et al. **Frequency of antibodies to *Erhlichia canis*, *Borrelia* burgdorferi and *Dirofilaria immitis* antigens in dogs in the Ilhéus-Itabuna micro-region, Bahia, Brazil.** Rev. Bras. Parasitol. Vet., v.16, n.3, p.117-120, 2007.

CARVALHO, F. S, et al. **Epidemiological and molecular study of Ehrlichia canis in dogs in Bahia, Brazil.** Genetics and Molecular Research, v.7, n.3, p. 657-662, 2008.

CASTRO-JUNIOR, G. et al. **Evidence Of *Leishmania (Leishmania) Infantum* Infection In Dogs From Juiz De Fora, Minas Gerais State, Brazil, Based On Immunochromatographic Dual-Path Platform (Dpp%) And Pcr Assays.** Rev. Ins. Med. Trop. São Paulo, v. 56, n. 3, p. 225-229, 2014.

CERON, E. P. **Characterisation and distribution of ticks in urban areas in the municipalities of Criciúma and Urussanga, southern Santa Catarina.** Research project - Universidade do Extremo Sul Catarinense (UNESC), Criciúma, Santa Catarina, 2014.

CONSTANTINO C.; et al. **Seroepidemiology of *Leishmania spp.* in dogs residing in Telêmaco Borba, Paraná, Brazil.** Agricultural Sciences, v. 35, n. 6, 2014.

COUTINHO, M. T. Z. et al. Participation of *Rhipicephalus sanguineus* (Acari: Ixodidae) in the epidemiology of canine visceral leishmaniasis. Vet Parasitol, v. 128, n. 1-2, p. 149-155, 2005.

DANTAS-TORRES, F. **Biology and ecology of the brown dog tick, *Rhipicephalus sanguineus*.** Parasites & Vectors, v. 3, n. 26, 2010.

DELL' PORTO A.; Oliveira, M.R.; Miguel, O. **Babesia canis in stray dogs of the city of São Paulo. Comparative studies between the clinical and haematological aspects and the indirect fluorescent antibody test.** Rev. Bras. Parasitol. Vet, v. 2, n.1, p. 37-40, 1993.

EPIDEMIOLOGICAL SURVEILLANCE DIRECTORATE. **Dive-SC participates in investigation of confirmed case of canine visceral leishmaniasis in Chapecó.** 2017. Available at : <http://www.dive.sc.gov.br/index.php/arquivo-noticias/587-dive-sc-participa-de-investigacaoo-de-caso-confirmado-de-leishmaniose-visceral-canina-em-chapeco>. Accessed on: 07 Sep. 2017.

DUMLER, J. S. et al. **Reorganisation of genera in the families *Rickettsiaceae* and *Anaplasmataceae* in the order *Rickettsiales*: unification of some species of *Ehrlichia* with *Anaplasma*, *Cowdria* with *Ehrlichia* and *Ehrlichia* with *Neorickettsia*, descriptions of six new species combinations and designation of *Ehrlichia equi and* HGE agent as subjective synonyms of *Ehrlichia phagocytophila*.** Int. J. Syst. Evolut. Microbiol., v. 51, p. 2145-2165, 2001.

FARIA, J. L. M.; RIBEIRO, S. C. A.; TINUCCI-COSTA, M. **Study of symptoms and changes in blood count and urinalysis in dogs with ehrlichiosis in the acute phase.** In: Congresso Brasileiro de Clínicos Veterinários de Pequenos Animais, 24, 2003, Belo Horizonte. Annals... Belo Horizonte: Congress, 2003. 1 CD-ROM.

FEITOSA, M. M. **Clinical evaluation of naturally infected animals. In: 1st Forum on Canine Visceral Leishmaniasis, 2006, Jaboticabal.** Proceedings... Jaboticabal: Colégio Brasileiro de Parasitologia Veterinária, Faculdade de Ciências Agrárias da Universidade Paulista, 2006, p. 9 - 14.

FIGUEIREDO, F. B. et al. **Canine Visceral Leishmaniasis: Two autochthonous cases in the municipality of Florianópolis, state of Santa Catarina.** Acta Scientiae Veterinariae, v. 40, n. 1, p. 1-4, 2012.

FONSECA, J.P; et al. Hematological Parameters and Seroprevalence of Ehrlichia canis and Babesia vogeli in Dogs. Ciência Animal Brasileira, v. 18, p. 1-9, 2017.

FREEMAN, M. J. et al. **Hypotensive shock syndrome associated with acute *Babesia canis* infection in a dog.** J. Am. Vet. Med. Assoc., v. 204, n. 1, p. 94-96, 1994.

FURUTA, P. I. et al. **Comparison between a soluble antigen-based ELISA and IFAT in detecting antibodies against *Babesia canis in* dogs.** Rev. Bras. Parasitol. Vet., v. 18, n. 3, p. 41-45, 2009.

GALLEGO, L. S. et al. **Directions for the diagnosis, clinical staging,** treatment and prevention of canine leishmaniosis.** Vet. Parasit., v. 165, p. 1-18, 2009.

GUIMARÃES, AM, et al. **Factors associated the seropositivity for *Babesia, Toxoplasma, Neospora* and *Leishmania* in dogs attended at nine veterinary clinics in the municipality of Lavras, MG.** Rev. Bras. Parasitol. Vet, v. 18. n. 1, p. 49-53, 2009.

HARRUS, S.; et al. **Molecular detection of *Ehrlichia canis, Anaplasma bovis, Anaplasma platys, Candidatus Midichloria mitochondrii* and *Babesia canis vogeli* in ticks from Israel.** Clin Microbiol Infect, v. 17, n.3, p. 459-463, 2011.

HARRUS, S. et al. **Amplification of ehrlichial DNA from dogs 34 months after infection with *Ehrlichia canis*.** J. Clin. Microbiol., v. 36, n. 1, p. 73-76, 1998.

HARRUS, S. et al. **Recent advances in determining the pathogenesis of canine monocytic ehrlichiosis.** J. Clin. Microbiol., v. 37, n. 9, p. 2745-2749, 1999.

HERNÁNDEZ, G. V. **Parasitological, molecular and serological detection of *Ehrlichia canis* and *Babesia canis* in dogs from the central-eastern region of Spain.**

Colombia. 2010, 76 p. Dissertation (Master's Degree)- Universidade Estadual Paulista, Jaboticabal- SP.

JACOBSON, N. L. S; CLARK, I. A. **The pathophysiology of canine

babesiosis: new approaches to an old puzzle. J. South Afr. Vet. Assoc., v. 65, p. 134-145, 1994.

KRAWCZAK, F.S.; et al. **Leishmania, *Babesia* and *Ehrlichia* in urban pet dogs: co-infection or cross-reaction in serological methods?** Revista da Sociedade Brasileira de Medicina Tropical, v. 48, n. 1, p. 64-68, 2015.

LABARTHE, N.; et al. **Serologic Prevalence of *Dirofilaria immitis, Ehrlichia canis,* and *Borrelia burgdorferi* Infections in Brazil**. Veterinary Therapeutics, v. 4, n. 1, p. 67-75, 2003.

LABRUNA, M. B.; PEREIRA, M. C. **Ticks in dogs in Brazil**. Clínica Veterinária, v. 30, p. 24-32, 2001.

LAPPIN, M. R. Protozoal and mixed infections. In: ETTINGER, S. J. & FELDMAN, E. C. **Treatise on veterinary internal medicine: diseases of the dog and cat**. 5. ed. Rio de Janeiro: Guanabara Koogan, 2004, p. 437 - 438.

LEWIS, G. E. **The brown dog tick *Rhipicephalus sanguineus* and the dog as experimental hosts of Ehrlichia *canis*.** Am. J. Vet. Res., v. 32, n. 12, p. 1953-1955, 1977.

MACINTIRE, D. K. et al. ***Babesia gibsoni* infection among dogs in the southeastern United States**. J. Am. Vet. Med. Assoc., v. 220, n. 3, p. 325329, 2002.

MARZOCHI, M. C. A. et al. **Visceral leishmaniasis in Rio de Janeiro, Brazil: eco-epidemiological aspects and control**. Rev. Soc. Bras. Med. Trop., v. 42, n. 5, p. 570-580, 2009.

MAZIERO, N.; et al. **Rural-urban focus of canine visceral leishmaniosis in the far werten region of Santa Catarina State, Brazil**. Vet Parasitol, v. 205, n. 1-2, p. 92-95, 2014.

MELO, Andréia L.T, et al. **Seroprevalence and risk factors to *Ehrlichia spp.* and *Rickettsia* spp. in dogs from the Pantanal Region of Mato Grosso State, Brazil.** Ticks and Tick-borne Diseases, v. 2, p. 213- 218, 2011.

MILKEN, V.M.F.; et al. **Occurrence of canine babesiosis in the municipality of Uberlândia, Minas Gerais**. Arq. Ciênc. Vet. Zool, v. 7, n. 1, p. 19-22, 2004.

MORAIS, A. N. et al. **Canine visceral leishmaniasis and Chagas disease among dogs in Araguaína, Tocantins).** Rev. Bras. Parasitol. Vet., v. 22, n. 2, p. 225 - 229, 2013.

NEER, T. M.; HARRUS, S. Canine ehrlichiosis. In: GREENE, C. E. **Infectious diseases of the dog and cat.** Third Edition, St. Louis: Saunders Elsevier, 2006. p. 203-232.

NELSON, R. W.; COUTO, C. G. **Small Animal Internal Medicine**. 3. ed. São Paulo: Elsevier Editora, 2006, 1324p.

O'DWYER, L.H.; et al. ***Babesia spp.* Infection in dogs from rural areas of São Paulo State, Brazil.** Rev. Bras. Parasitol. Vet, v. 18, n. 2, p. 23-26, 2009.

OLIVEIRA, D. et al. **Anti-Ehrlichia *canis* antibodies detection by "Dot-ELISA" in naturally infected dogs.** Rev. Bras. Parasitol. Vet., v. 9, n. 1, p. 1-5, 2000.

PASSOS, V.M., et al. **Natural infection of a domestic cat (*Felis domesticus*) with *Leishmania* (Viannia) in the metropolitan region of Belo Horizonte, State of Minas Gerais, Brazil**. Mem. Inst. Oswaldo Cruz, v. 91, p.19-20, 1996.

PENAFORTE, K. M. et al. **Leishmania infection in a population of dogs: an epidemiological investigation relating to visceral leishmaniasis control**. Rev. Bras. Parasitol. Vet., v. 22, n. 4, p. 592-596, 2013.

PEREGO, R.; et al. **Prevalence of Dermatological Presentations of Canine Leishmaniasis in a Nonendemic Area: A Retrospective Study of 100 Dogs**. Hindawi Publishing Corporation Veterinary Medicine International, v. 2014, 5 p, 2014.

PINTO, R. L. **Babesiosis canina - Case report**. Monograph- Department of Animal Sciences, Federal Rural University of the Semi-Arid, Mossoró, Rio Grande do Norte, 2009.

FLORIANÓPOLIS CITY HALL. **Capital registers first case of human visceral leishmaniasis.** 2017. Available at: <http://www.pmf.sc.gov.br/entidades/saude/?pagina=notpagina&menu=3¬i=18752>. Accessed on: 04 Sep. 2017.

RAMOS, R.; et al. **Molecular survey and genetic characterisation of tick-borne pathogens in dogs in metropolitan Recife (north-eastern Brazil).** Parasitol Res, v. 107, n.5, p. 1115-1120, 2010.

SAITO, T. B.; et al. **Canine Infection by *Rickettsiae* and *Ehrlichiae* in Southern Brazil.** Am. J. Trop. Med. Hyg., v. 79, n. 1, p. 102 - 108, 2008.

SILVA, A. B., et al. **Molecular detection of *Babesia canis vogeli* in dogs and *Rhipicephalus sanguineus* in the mesoregion of western Maranhão, northeastern Brazil**. Ci Anim Bras, v. 13, n. 3, p. 388-395, 2012.

SILVA, C. B. S.; et al. **Seroepidemiological aspects of *Leishmania* spp. in dogs in the Itaguai micro-region, Rio de Janeiro, Brazil**. Rev. Bras. Parasit. Vet., v. 22, n. 1, p. 39-45, 2013.

SILVA, F. S. **Pathology and pathogenesis of canine visceral leishmaniasis**. Rev. Trop. - Ciências Agrárias e Biológicas, v. 1, n. 1, p. 20-31, 2007.

SILVA, I. P. M. **Canine ehrlichiosis - Literature review.** Scientific Journal of Veterinary Medicine. Year XIII-Number 24 - January 2015.

SOUSA, K. C. M. **Co-infection by *Erlichia canis, Leishmania chagasi* and *Babesia canis* in naturally infected dogs in Campo Grande, Mato Grosso do Sul.** Master's thesis - Faculty of Agricultural and Veterinary Sciences - UNESP. Jaboticabal, São Paulo, 2012.

TABOADA, J.; LOBETTI, R. Canine Babesiosis. In: GREENE, C. E. **Infectious Diseases of the dog and cat.** 3ed. Philadelphia : W. B Saunders, 2006, p. 722 - 735.

TOMAZ-SOCCOL, V. et al. **Allochthonous cases of canine visceral leishmaniasis in Paraná, Brazil: epidemiological implications**. Rev. Bras. Parasit. Vet., v. 18, n. 3, p. 46 - 51, 2009.

TRAPP, S.M.; et al. **Seroepidemiology of canine babesiosis and** ehrlichiosis in a hospital population. Vet. Parasitol, v.140, n. 3-4, p. 223230, 2006.

VARGAS HERNANDEZ, G. **Parasitological, molecular and serological detection of *Ehrlichia canis* and *Babesia canis* in dogs from the central-eastern region of Colombia.** Master's Degree - Faculty of Agricultural and Veterinary Sciences - UNESP. Jaboticabal, São Paulo, 2010.

VARGAS-HERNÁNDEZ, G.; et al. **Molecular and serological detection of *Ehrlichia canis* and *Babesia vogeli* in dogs in Colombia.** Vet Parasitol, v. 186, n. 3-4, p. 254-260, 2012.

VIEIRA, T. S. W. J. et al. **Serosurvey of tick-borne pathogens in dogs from urban and rural areas of Parana State, Brazil.** Rev. Bras. Parasitol. Vet., v. 22, n. 1, p. 104-109, 2013.

VILELA, JAR, et al. **Clinical and haematological changes in *Babesia canis vogeli* infection in dogs from the municipality of Seropédica, Rio de Janeiro, Brazil.** Rev. Bras. Med. Vet., v. 35, n. 1, p. 63-68, 2013.

VIOL, M. A., et al. **Identification of *Leishmania* spp. promastigotes in the intestines, ovaries, and salivary glands of *Rhipicephalus sanguineus* actively infesting dogs.** Parasitol Res, v. 115, n. 9, p. 3479-3484, 2016.

WANER, T. et al. **Canine Monocytic Ehrlichiosis - an overview.** Isr. J. Vet. Med., v. 54, n. 4, p. 103-107, 1999.

WANER, T. et al. **Characterisation of subclinical phase of canine ehrlichiosis in experimentally infected beagles dogs.** Vet. Parasitol., v. 69,

p. 307-317, 1997.

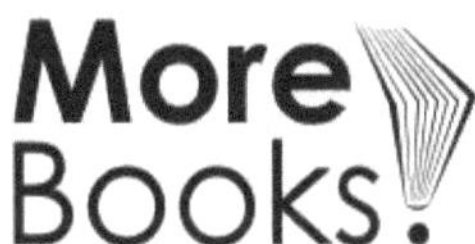

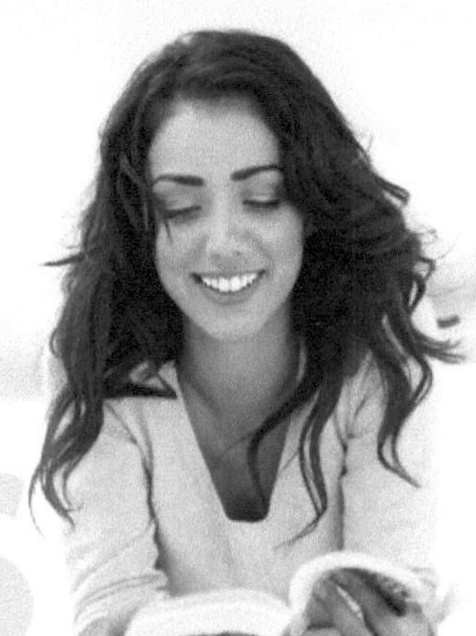

I want morebooks!

Buy your books fast and straightforward online - at one of world's fastest growing online book stores! Environmentally sound due to Print-on-Demand technologies.

Buy your books online at
www.morebooks.shop

Kaufen Sie Ihre Bücher schnell und unkompliziert online – auf einer der am schnellsten wachsenden Buchhandelsplattformen weltweit! Dank Print-On-Demand umwelt- und ressourcenschonend produzi ert.

Bücher schneller online kaufen
www.morebooks.shop

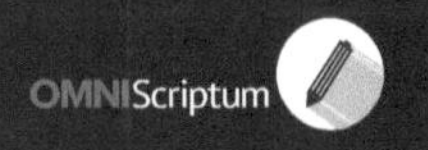

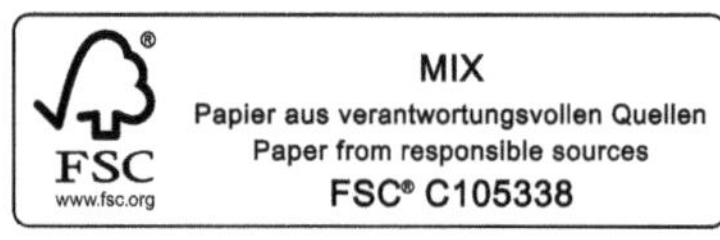